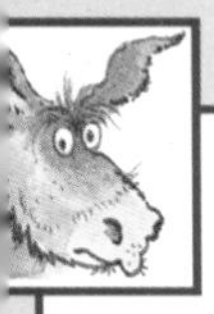
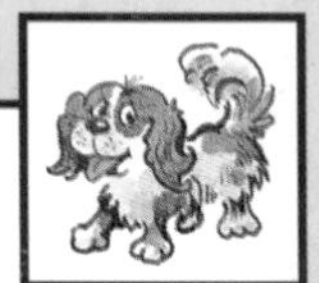

The Donkey and the Lapdog

and

The Lion and the Mouse

by Val Biro

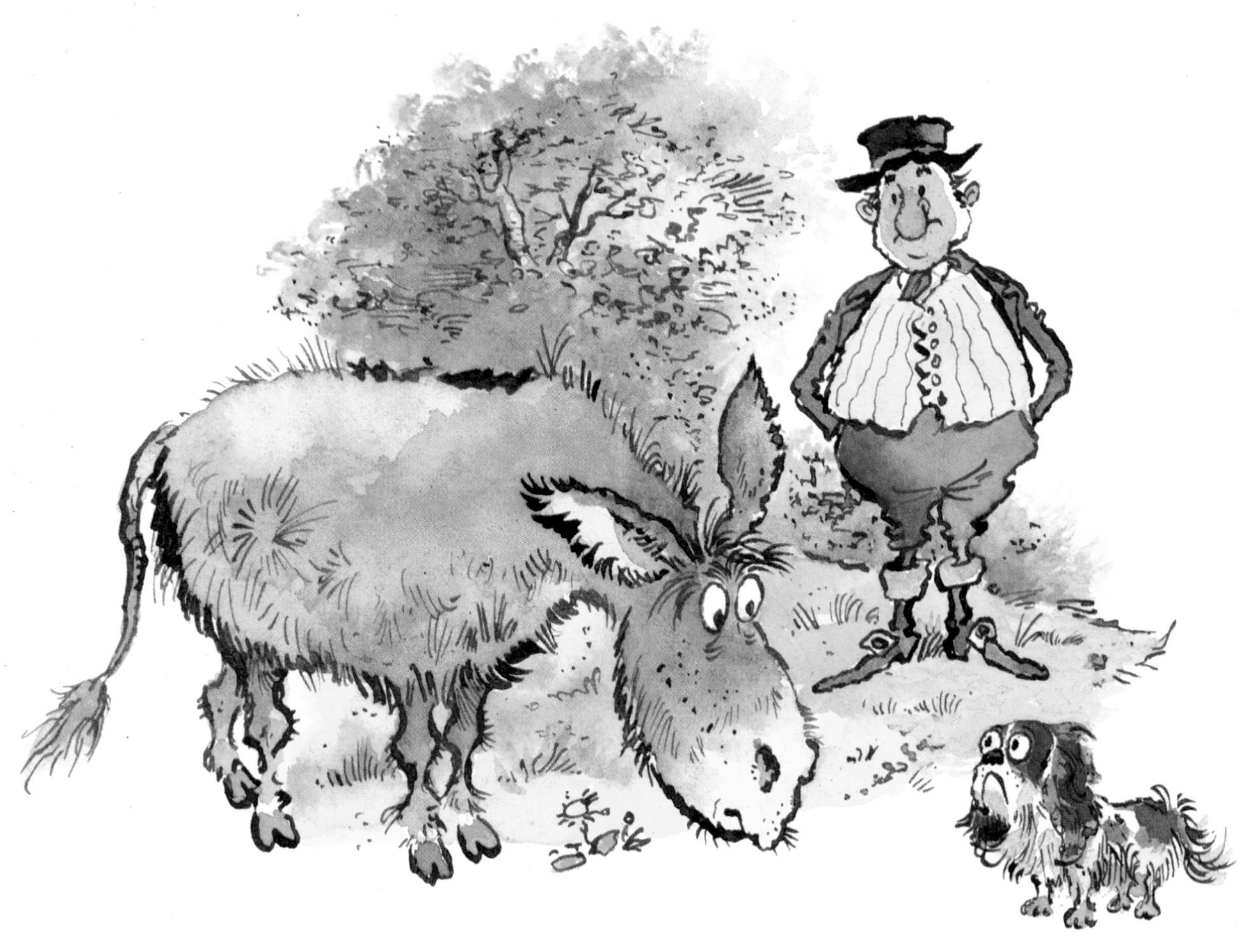

AWARD PUBLICATIONS LIMITED

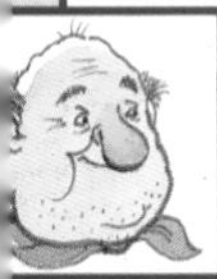
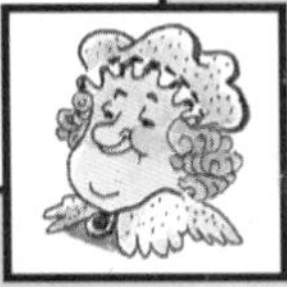

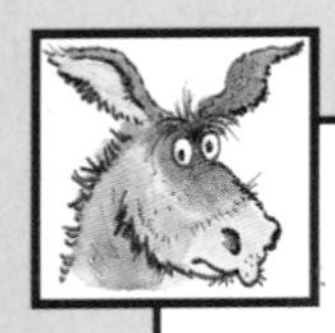

Once there was a man who had a house and a farm.

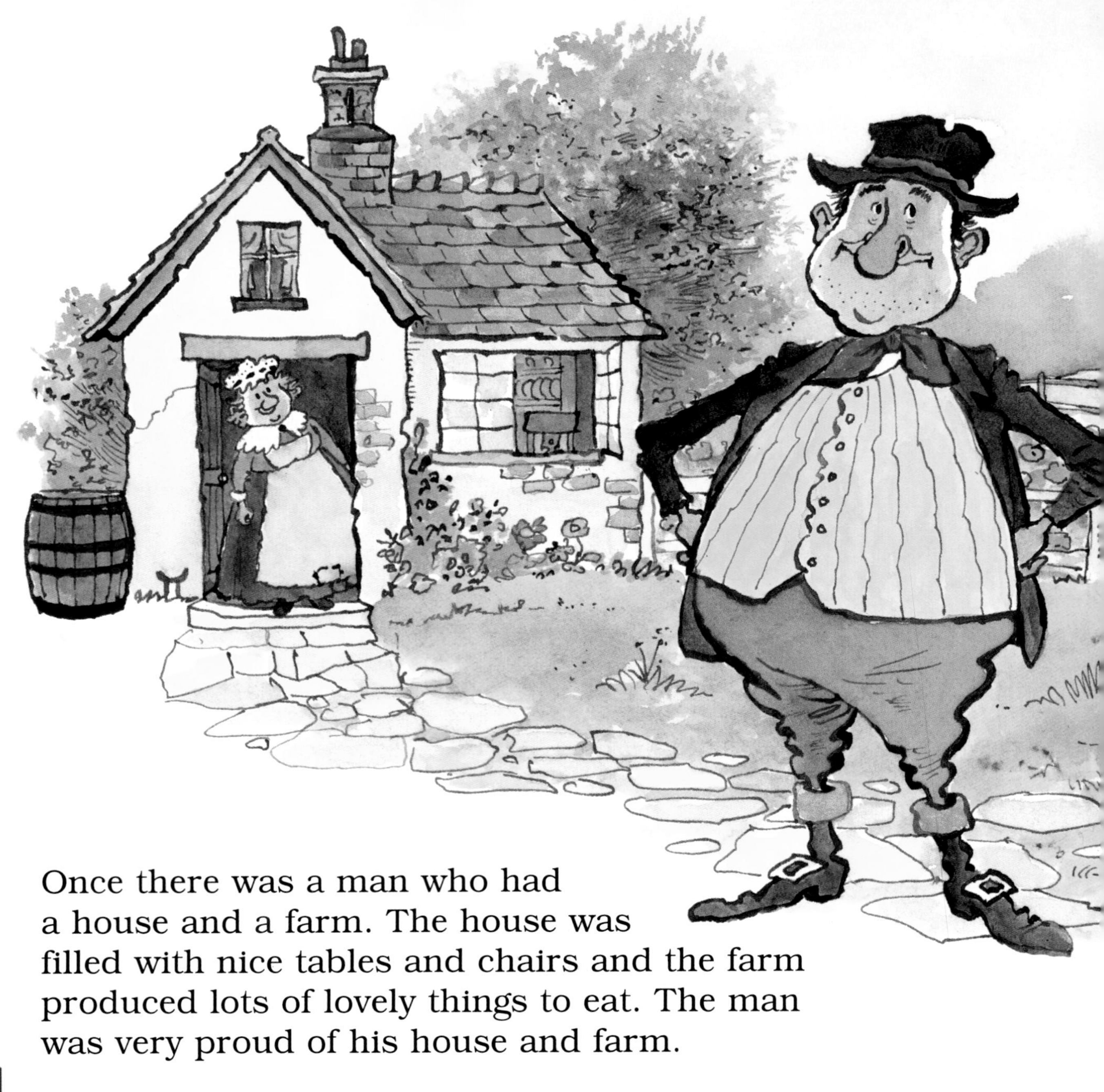

Once there was a man who had a house and a farm. The house was filled with nice tables and chairs and the farm produced lots of lovely things to eat. The man was very proud of his house and farm.

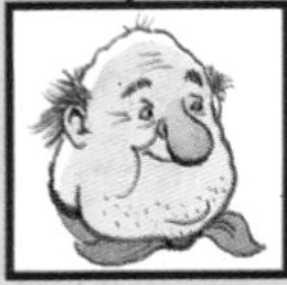

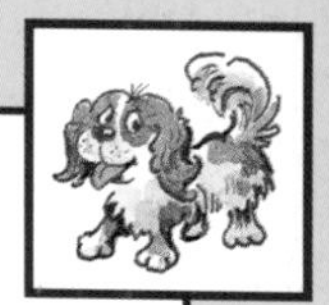

He also had a donkey and a lapdog.

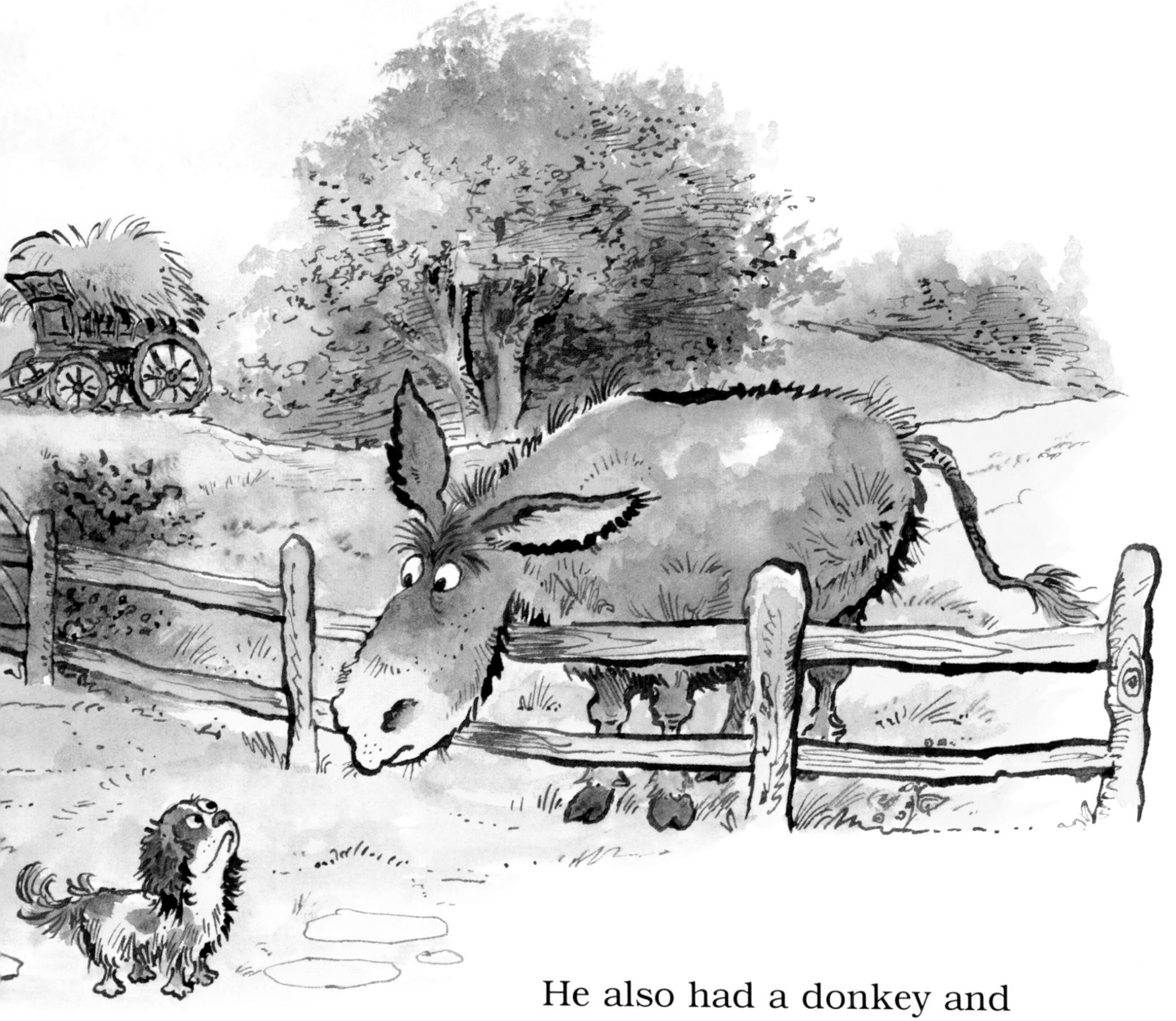

He also had a donkey and a lapdog. Both animals had four legs, but otherwise they were very different.

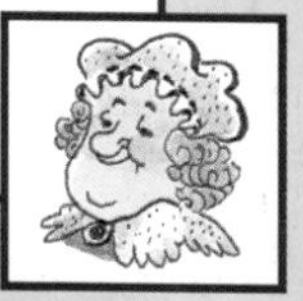

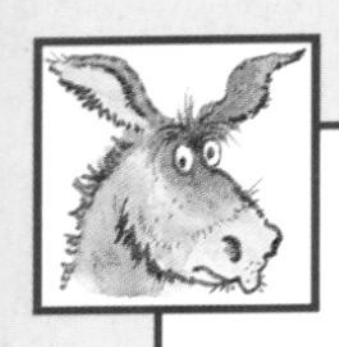
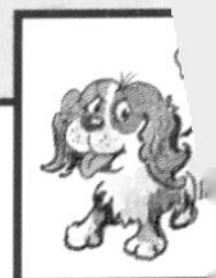

The donkey worked hard all day on the farm and he slept in the stable at night.

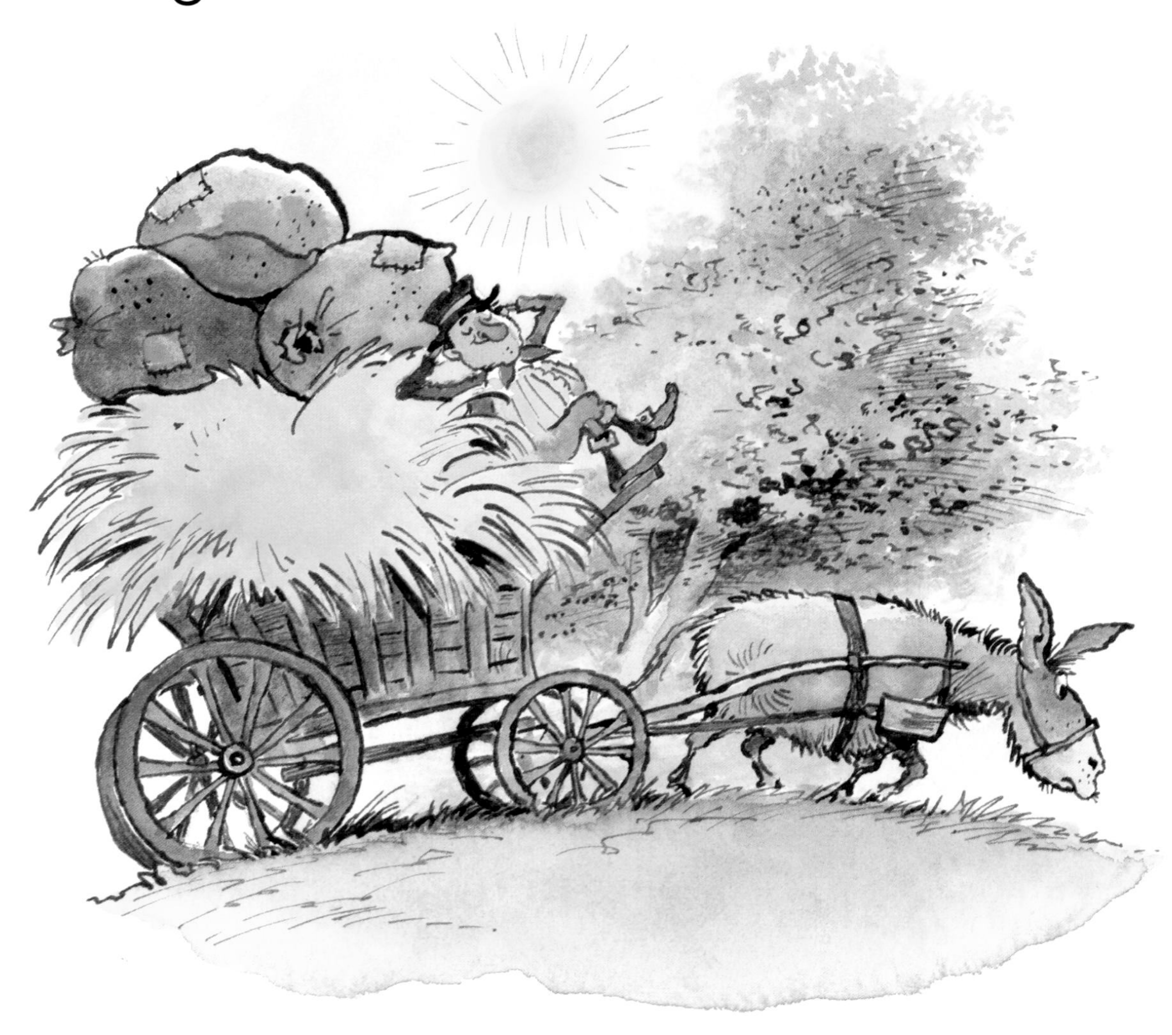

The donkey worked hard all day on the farm. He was very good at it. He always had plenty of food and he slept in the stable at night.

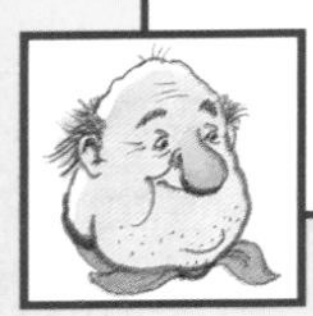
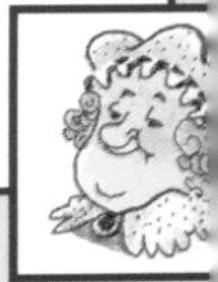

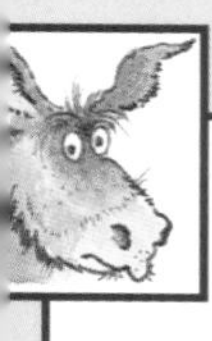
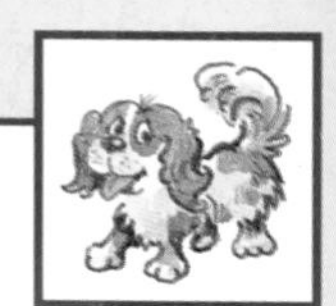

"Look at me," he said, "carting and carrying all day long while that silly dog has an easy life."

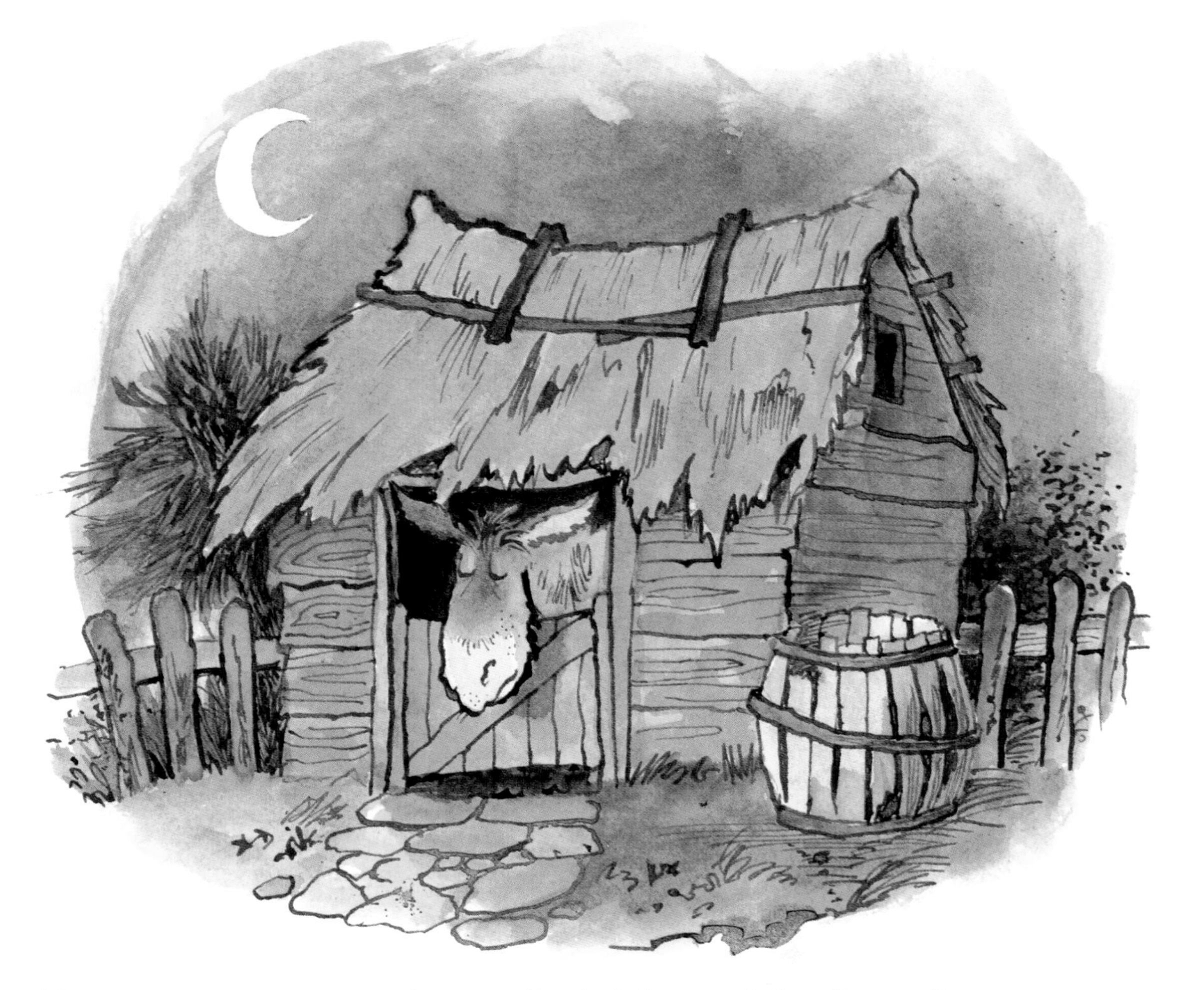

It was a warm and comfortable stable, but the donkey kept thinking about the lapdog.

"I cart and carry all day long," he said to himself, "while that silly dog has an easy life with everybody making a fuss of him!"

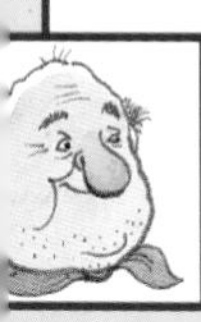
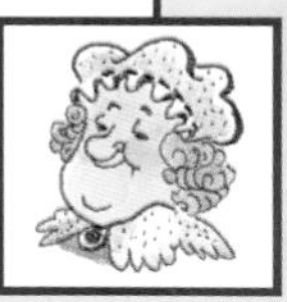

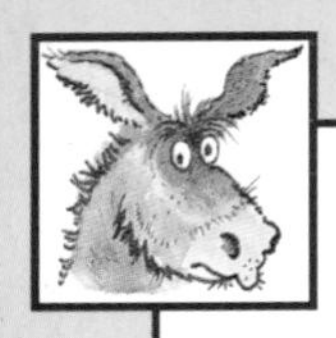
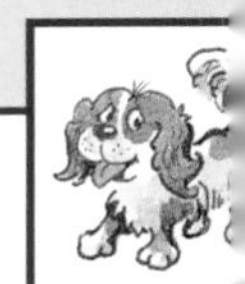

The lapdog played all day in the house . . .

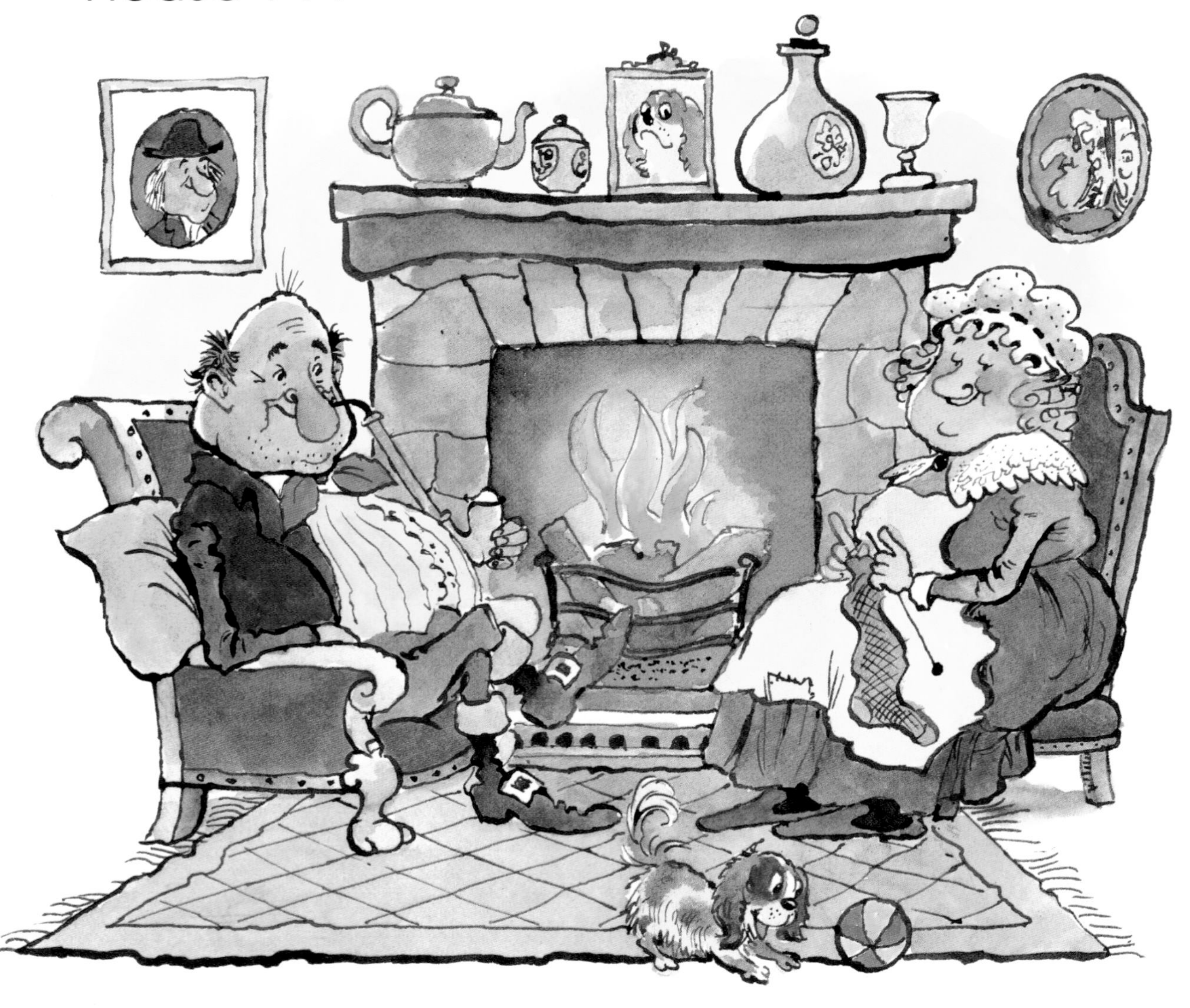

This was perfectly true because the lapdog played all day in the house, and he was very good at it. So good, in fact, that everybody fussed over and petted him and he didn't do a stroke of work.

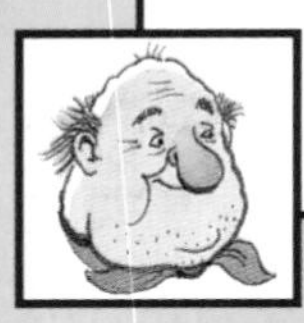
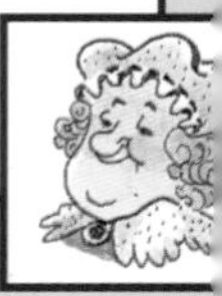

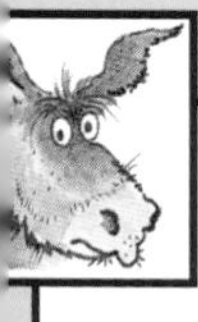
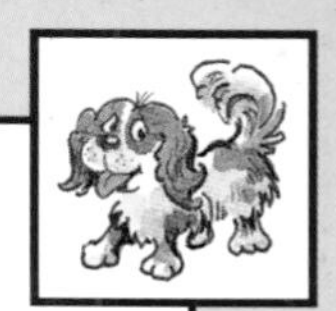

. . . and he slept in a soft bed at night.

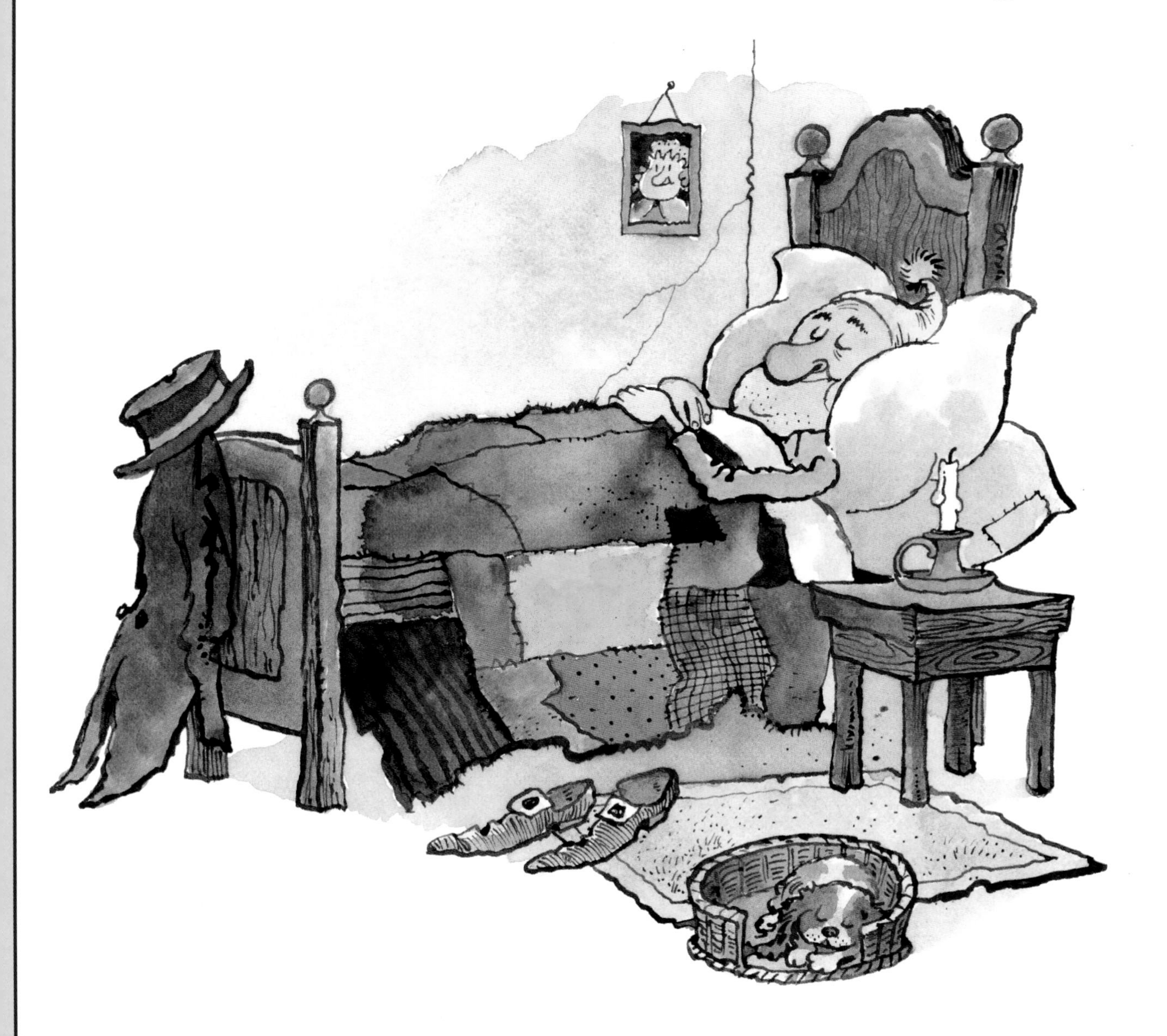

He just enjoyed himself all day and he slept in a soft bed at night, a real doggy bed, right by the side of his master.

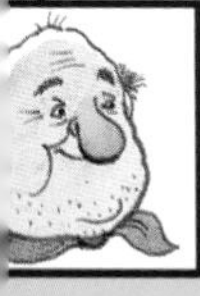
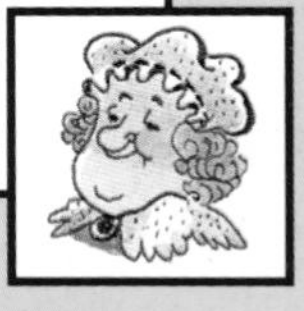

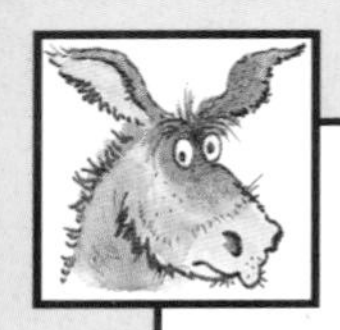

He sat on his master's lap at dinner and he had lovely things to eat. The donkey looked through the window and he was very jealous.

At mealtimes he would do what he could do best of all; he would sit on people's laps. That's why he was called a lapdog. He sat on his master's lap at dinner, and he had lovely things to eat. What a lucky dog!

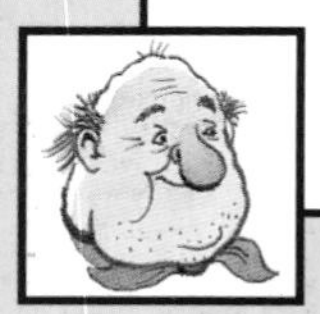

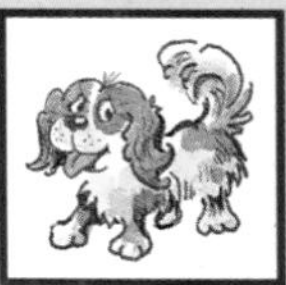

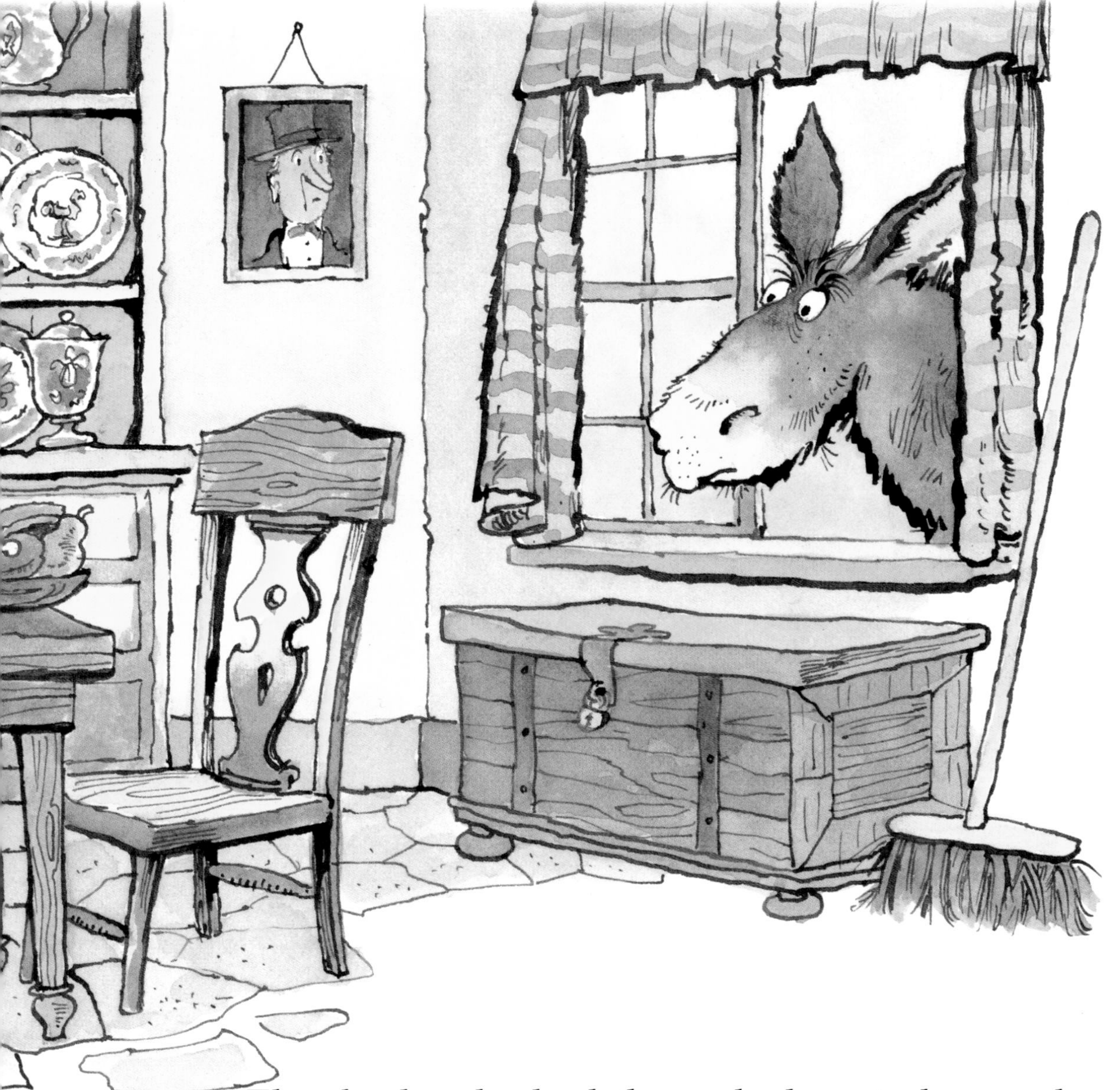

The donkey looked through the window and he was very jealous.

"That dog must be very clever," he thought, "to have all that fussing and petting and all that lovely food without having to do any work for it."

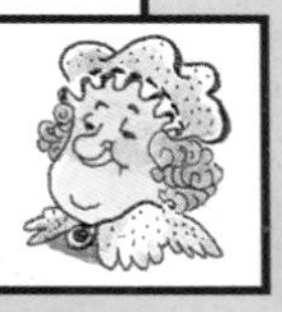

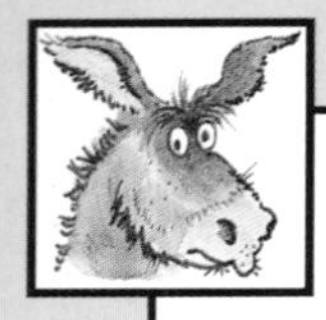

So one day he trotted into the house and began to play just like the dog.

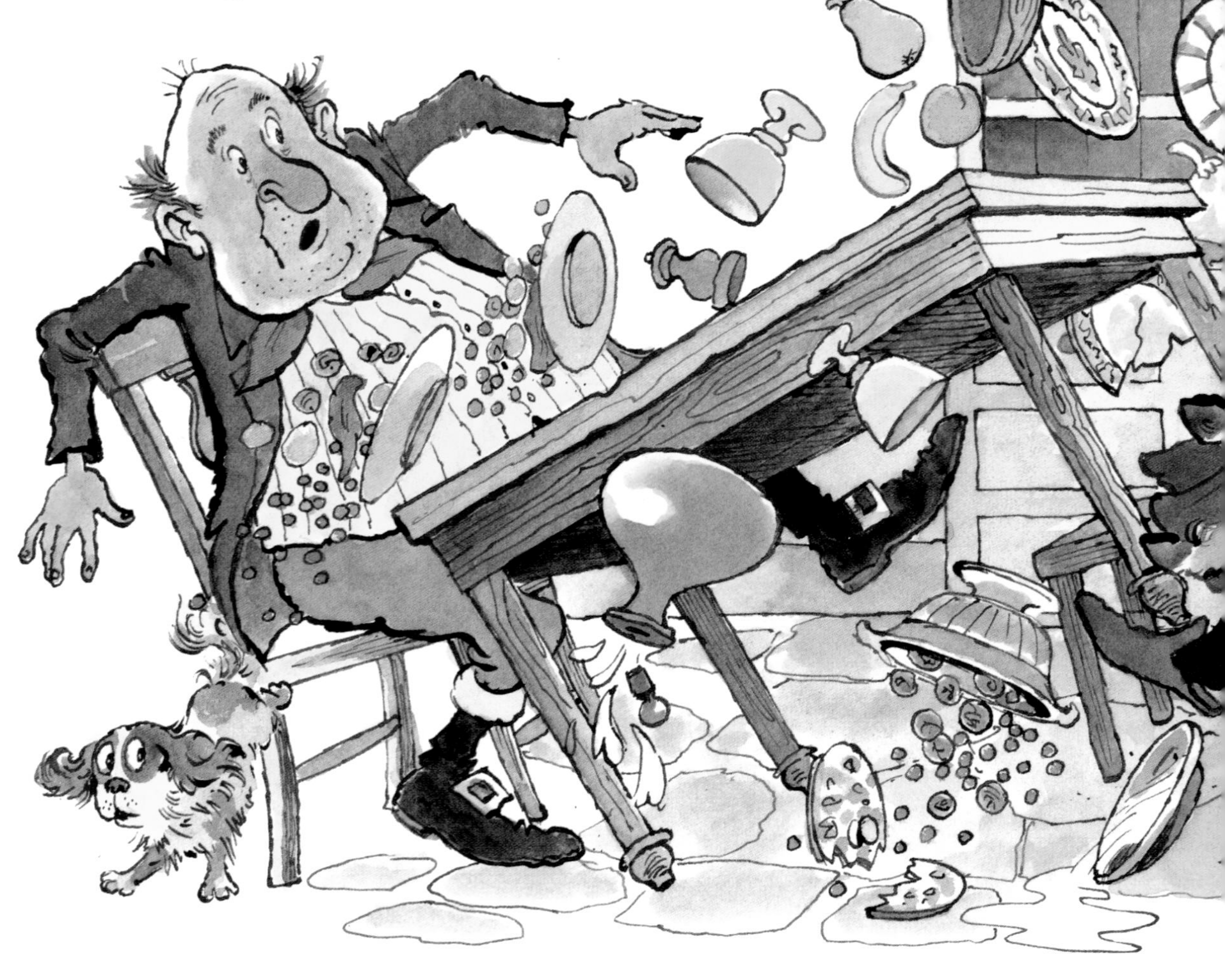

The donkey said, "I wish I could be more like the dog. The farmer and his wife would make a pet of me and I would do nothing but play all day."

So one day he trotted into the house and began to play just like the dog.

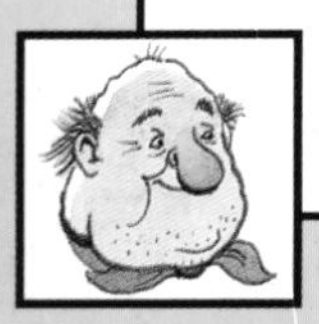

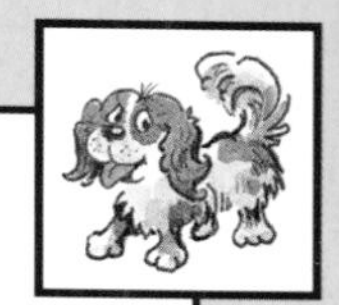

But he upset the tables and chairs!

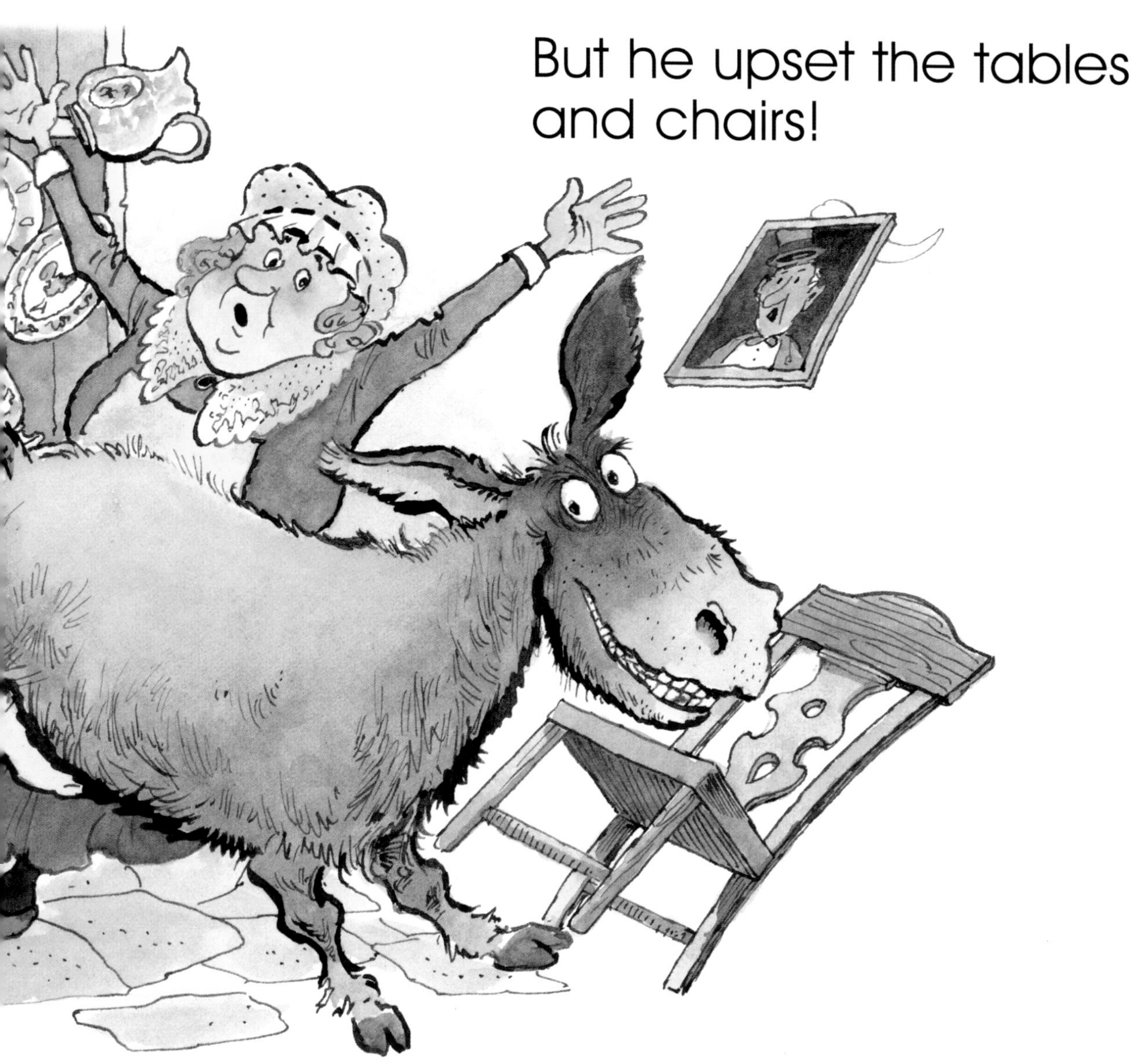

He jumped and capered around the room, but he upset the table and chairs. He was far too big and clumsy. Soon the room was a mess.

"Never mind!" the donkey thought and he tried to bark just like the little lapdog, but all he could say was "HEE-HAW!"

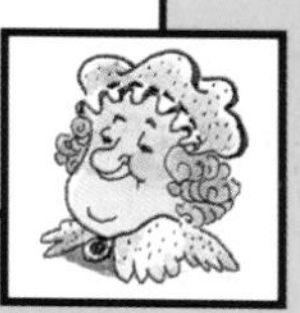

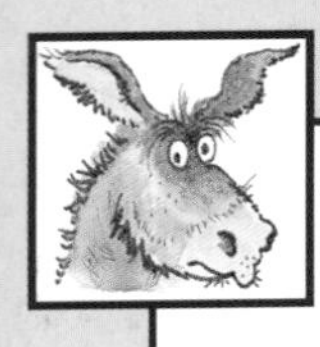

Then he saw the
lovely things to eat.
He jumped up on
his master's lap,
just like the
dog.

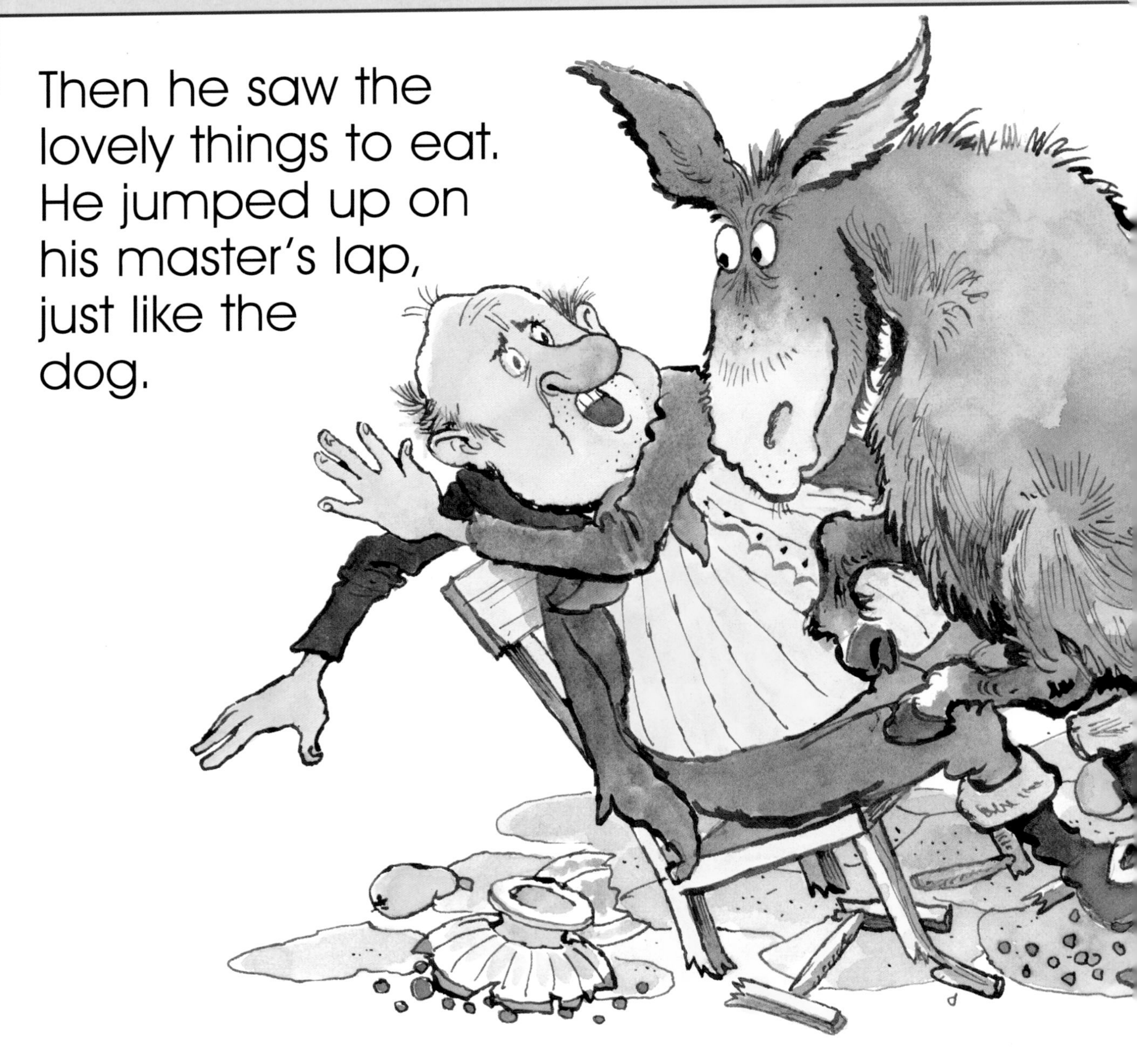

Then he saw the lovely things to eat. He jumped up on his master's lap, just like the dog.

"That should do the trick," thought the donkey.

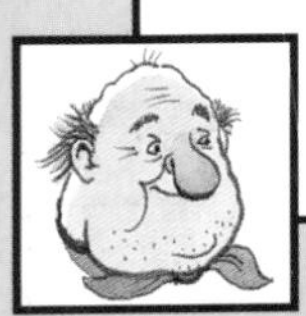

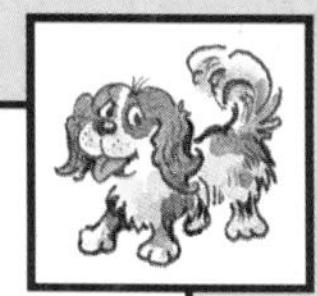

The master was very angry.

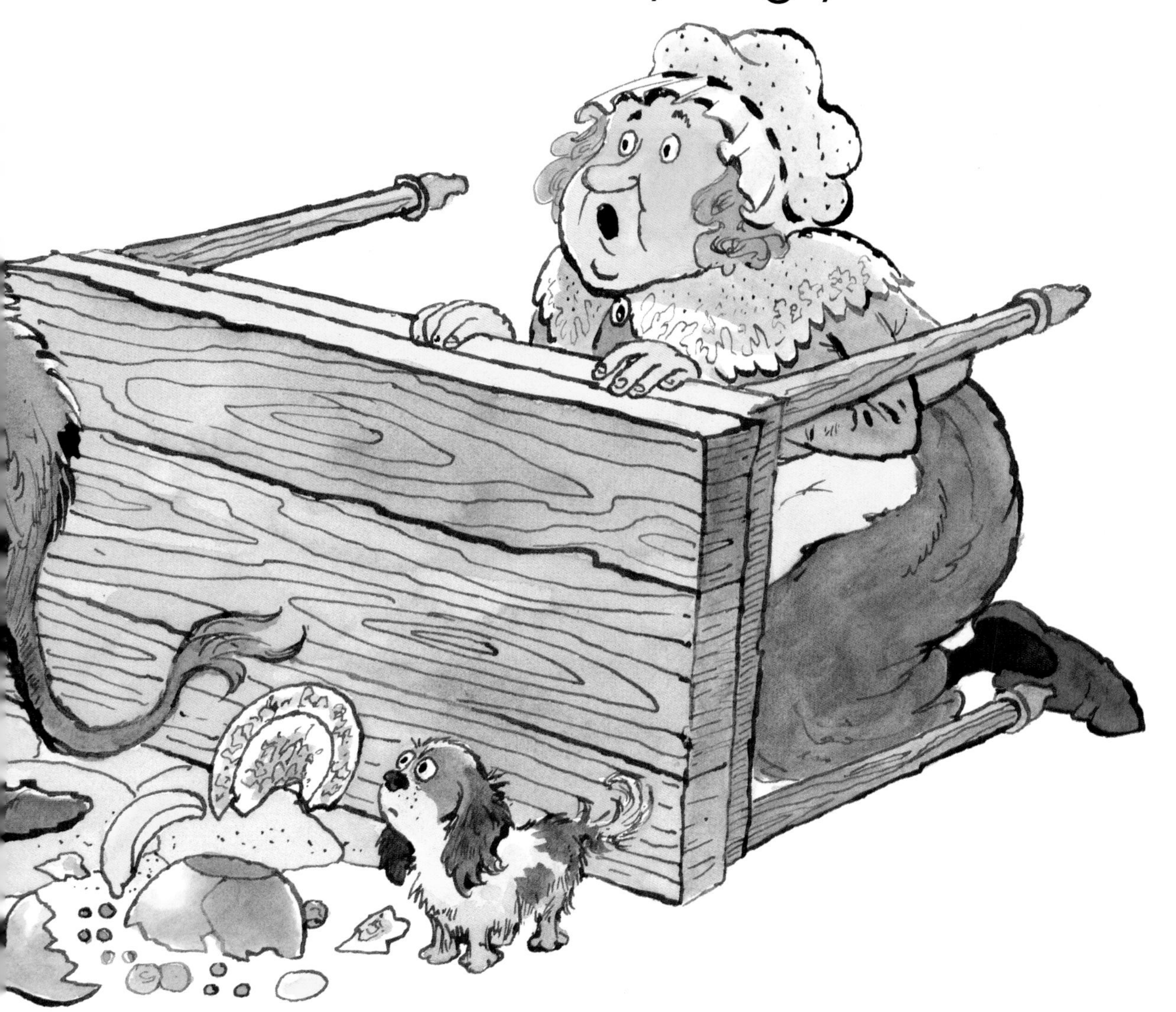

"Now my master will fuss over me and pet me and give me lovely food for being such a good lapdog."

But not a bit of it. The master was very angry. He jumped up, shouting, "You clumsy brute! What do you think you are doing? You're a donkey, not a lapdog!"

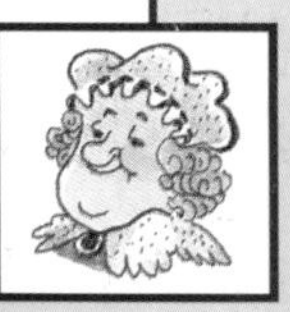

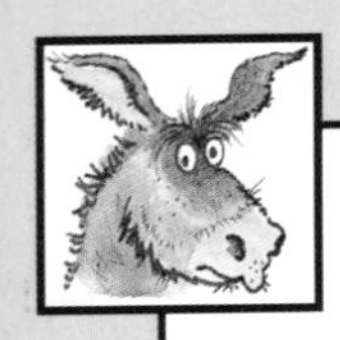

He grabbed a broom and chased the donkey back to the stable.

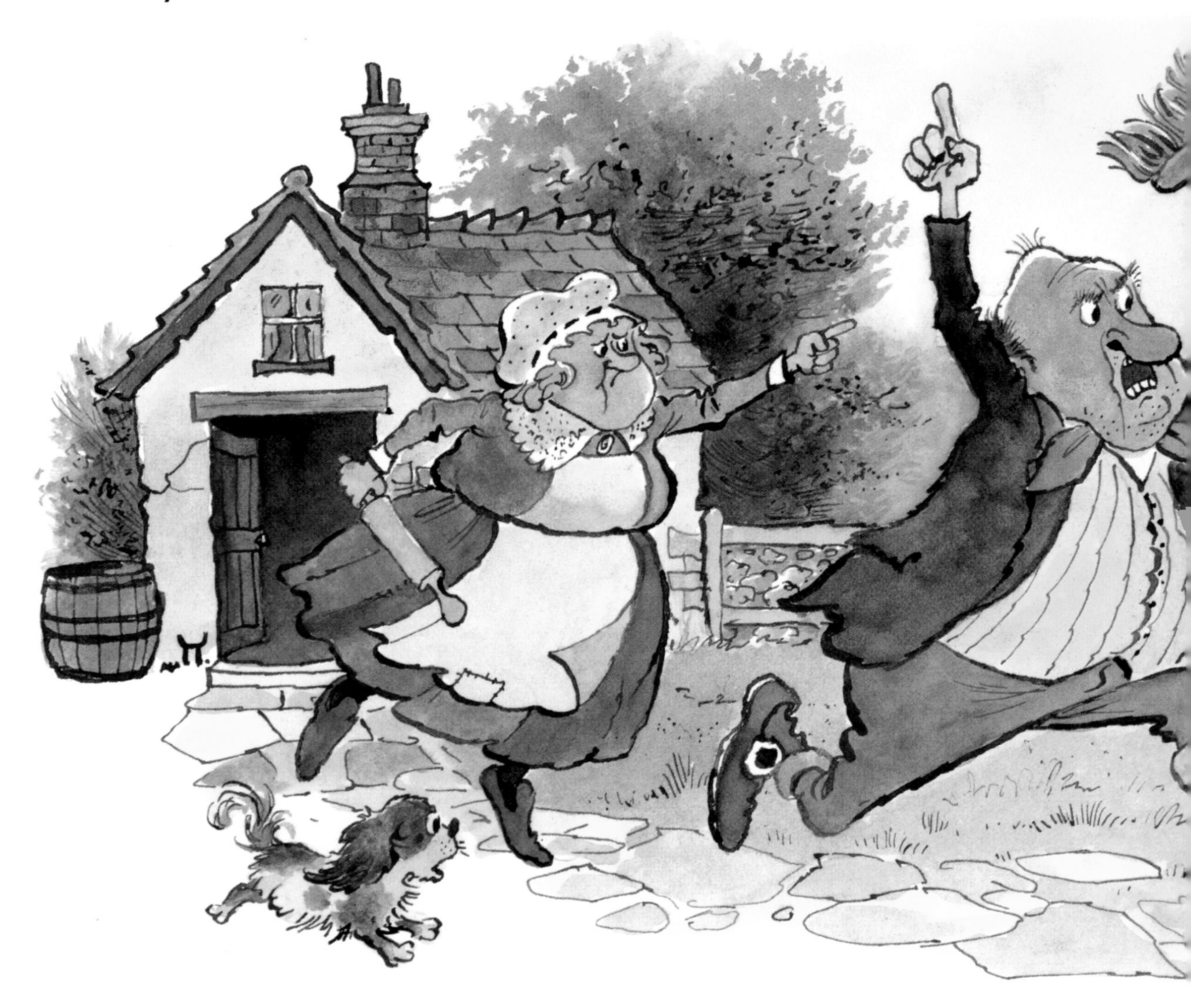

He grabbed a broom and chased the donkey back to the stable. The master's wife ran after the donkey and the master, shaking her rolling-pin, and the lapdog ran after them all!

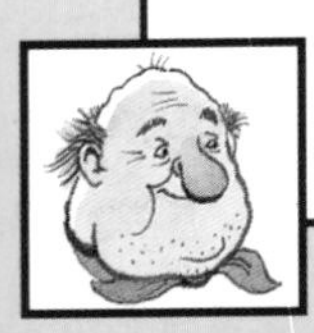

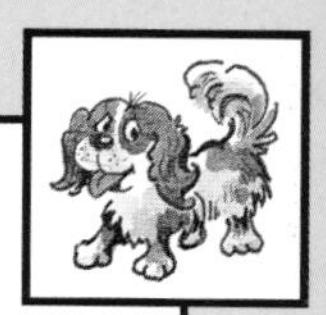

"HEE-HAW, HEE-HAW!" brayed the donkey as he ran back to his stable.

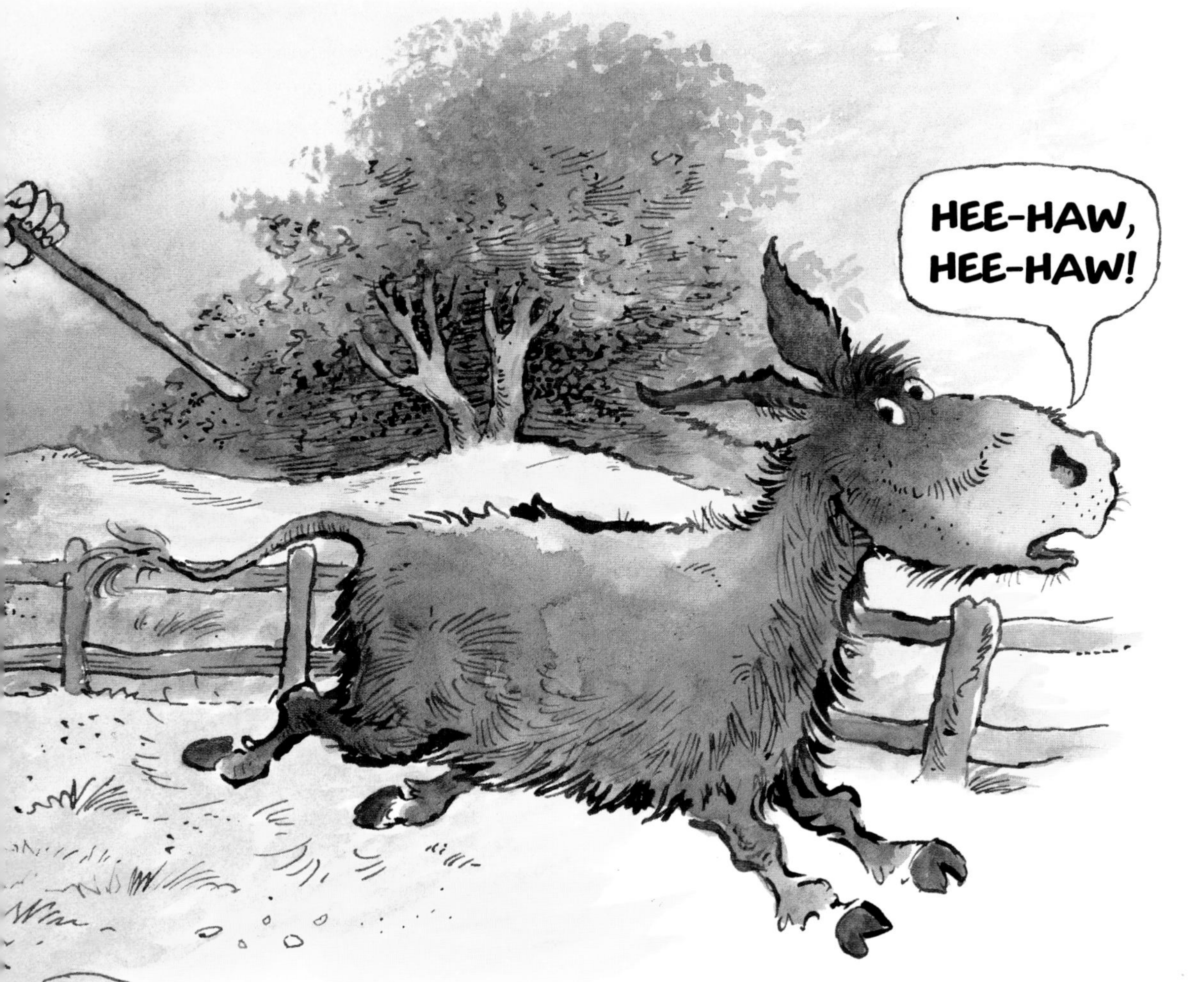

"HEE-HAW, HEE-HAW!" brayed the donkey as he ran back to his stable.

The donkey decided he had been silly to pretend to be a lapdog. Lapdogs were silly and useless. It was better to be a donkey, doing donkey work, eating donkey food, and sleeping in a donkey stable.

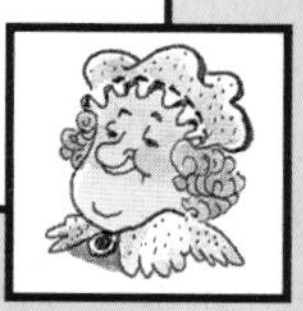

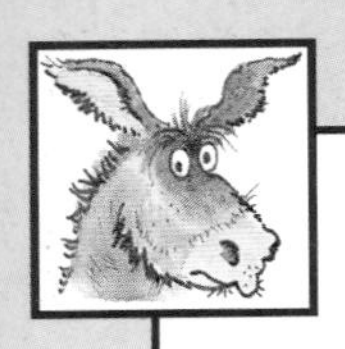
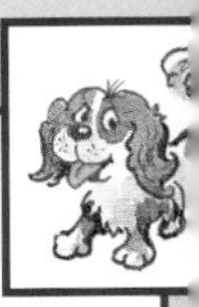

"I am no good at being a lapdog," said the donkey. "I will just be a donkey."

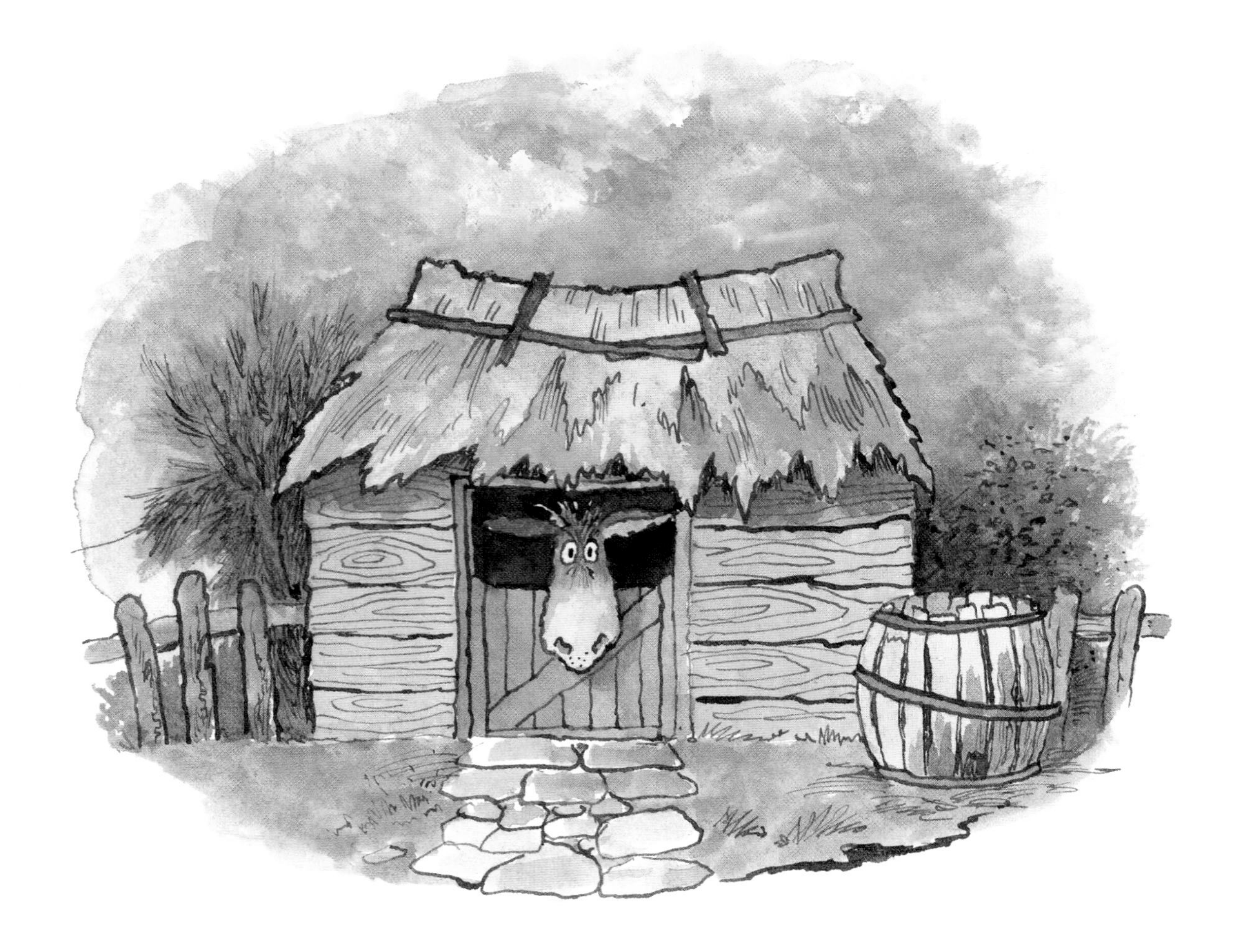

"I am no good at being a lapdog," said the donkey. "I will just be a donkey."

And he has been a donkey ever since, which is what he had been best at being all along.

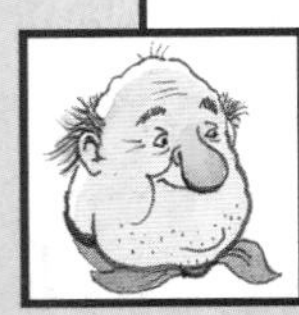
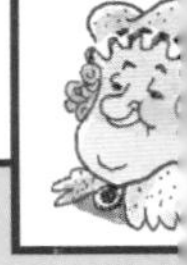

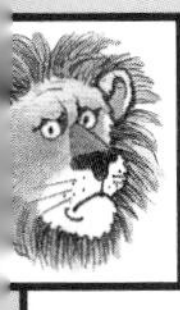
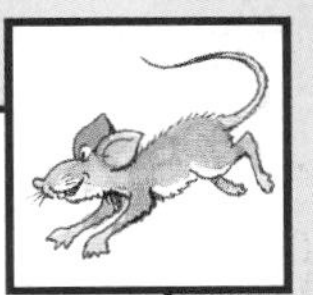

The Lion and the Mouse

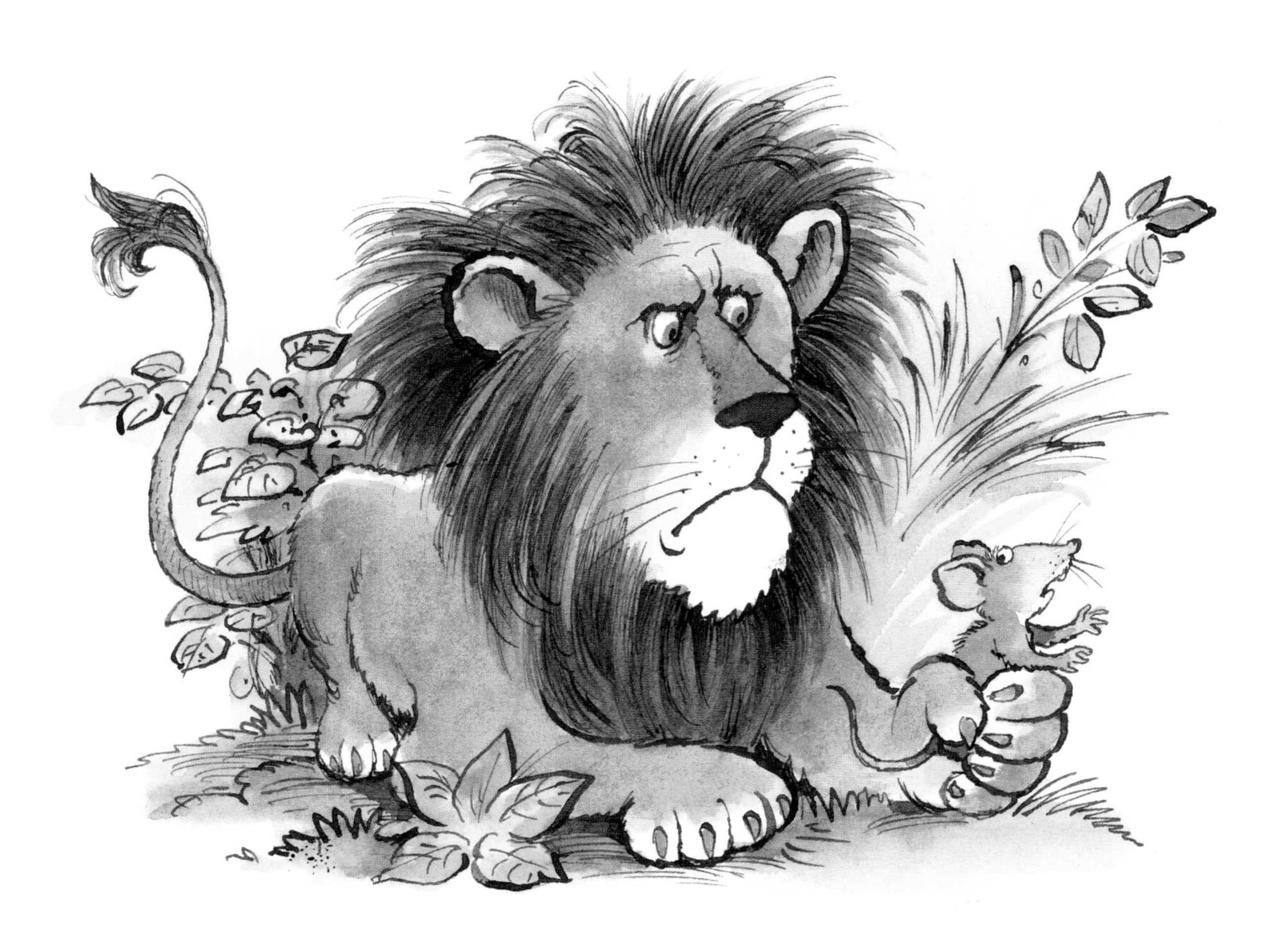

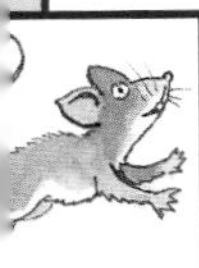
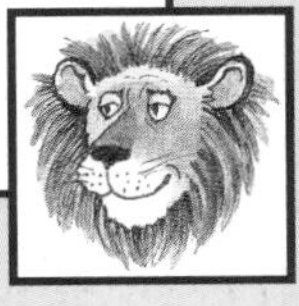

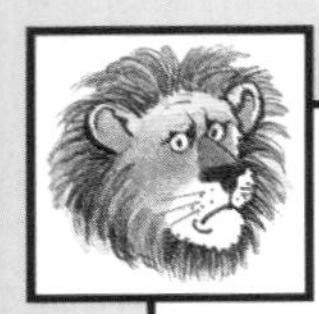

Once a lion caught a mouse.
He wanted to eat it.

Once a lion caught a mouse. He wanted to eat it.

"This mouse is so small it will never make me a meal," said the lion, "but I might as well gobble it up."

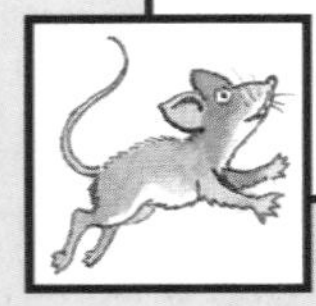

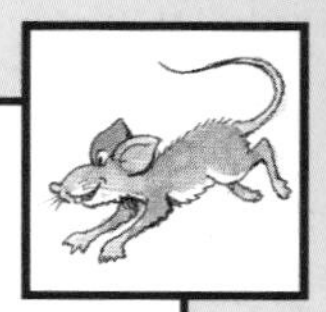

"Please let me go!" cried the mouse. "Be kind to me and one day I will help you."

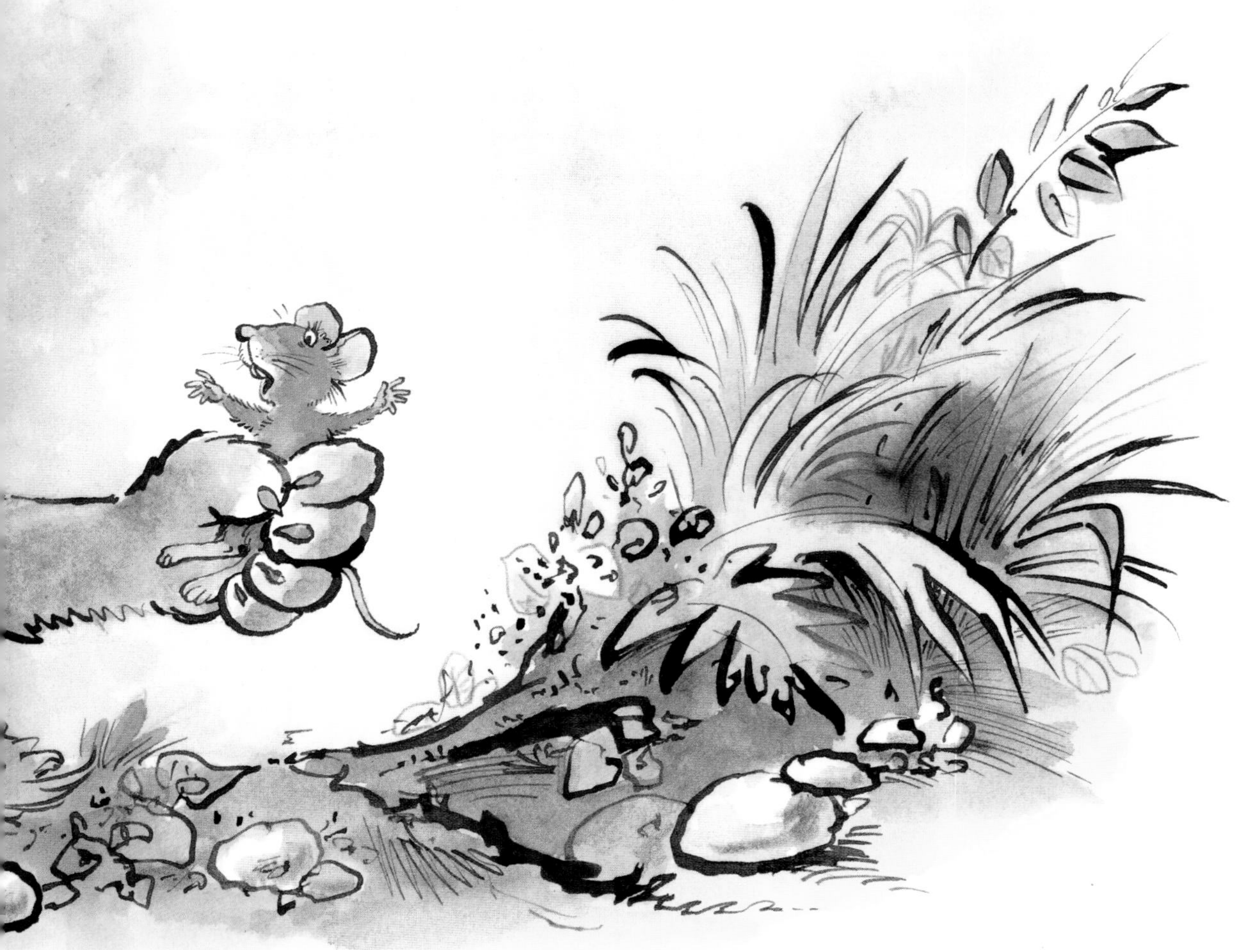

"Please let me go!" cried the mouse. "Be kind to me and one day I will help you." That was a funny thing to say because how could a tiny mouse ever help a big strong lion? It sounded ridiculous!

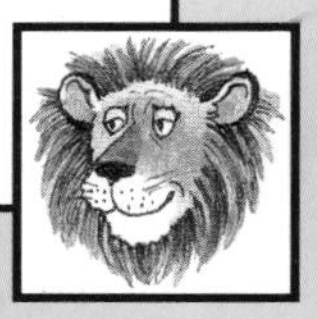

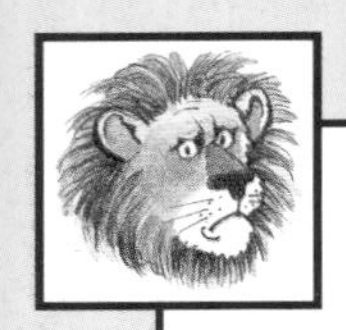
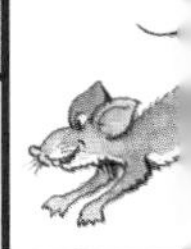

The lion laughed. "How could a little mouse ever help *me*?" But he let the mouse go.

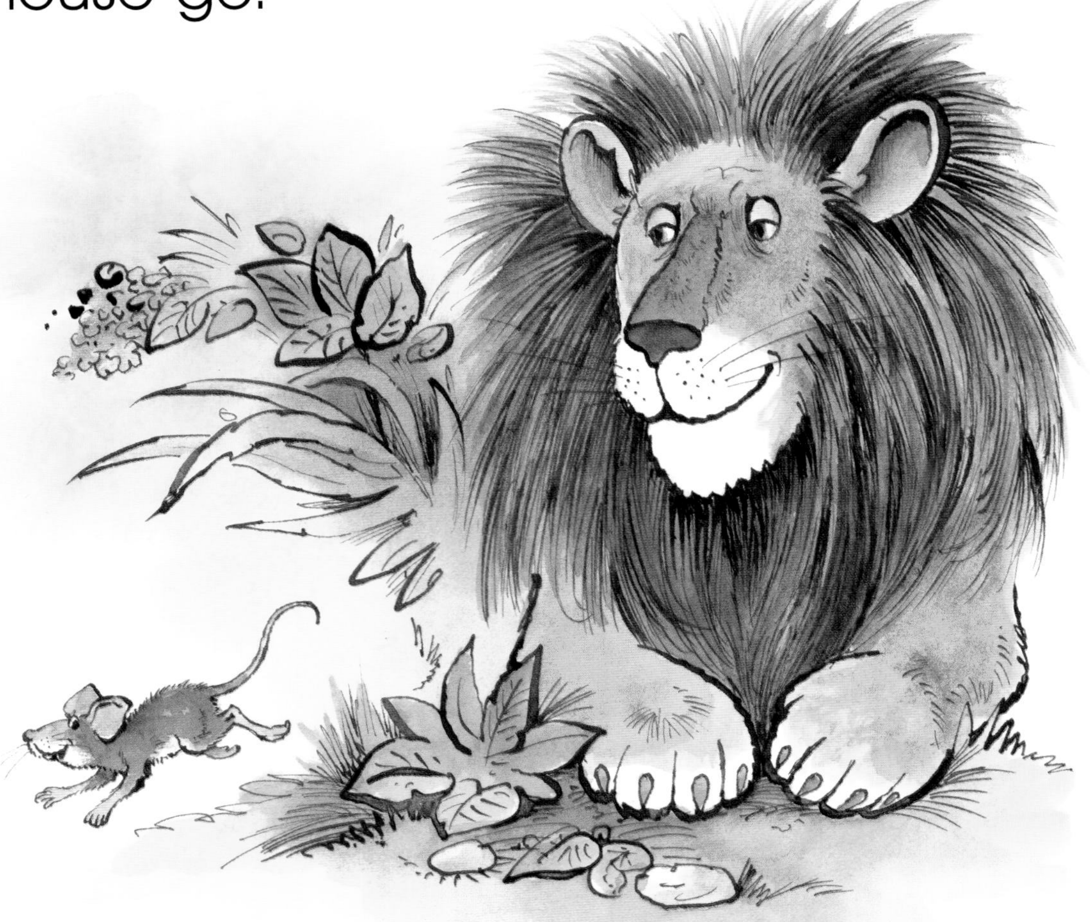

The lion laughed. "How could a little mouse ever help *me*?" But he let the mouse go because the mouse was brave enough to speak to him. Besides, the lion wasn't very hungry anyway. The mouse squeaked his thanks and scampered away.

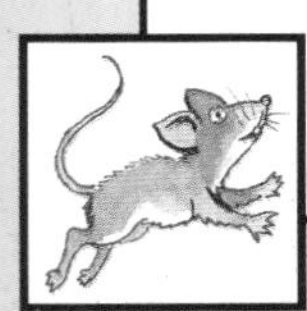
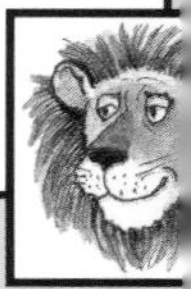

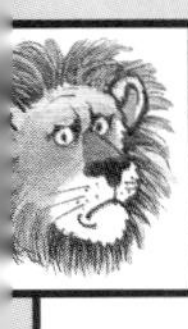
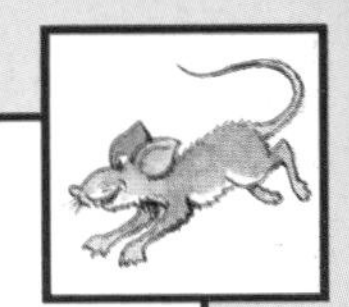

Soon after, the lion was caught in a net. He roared with anger.

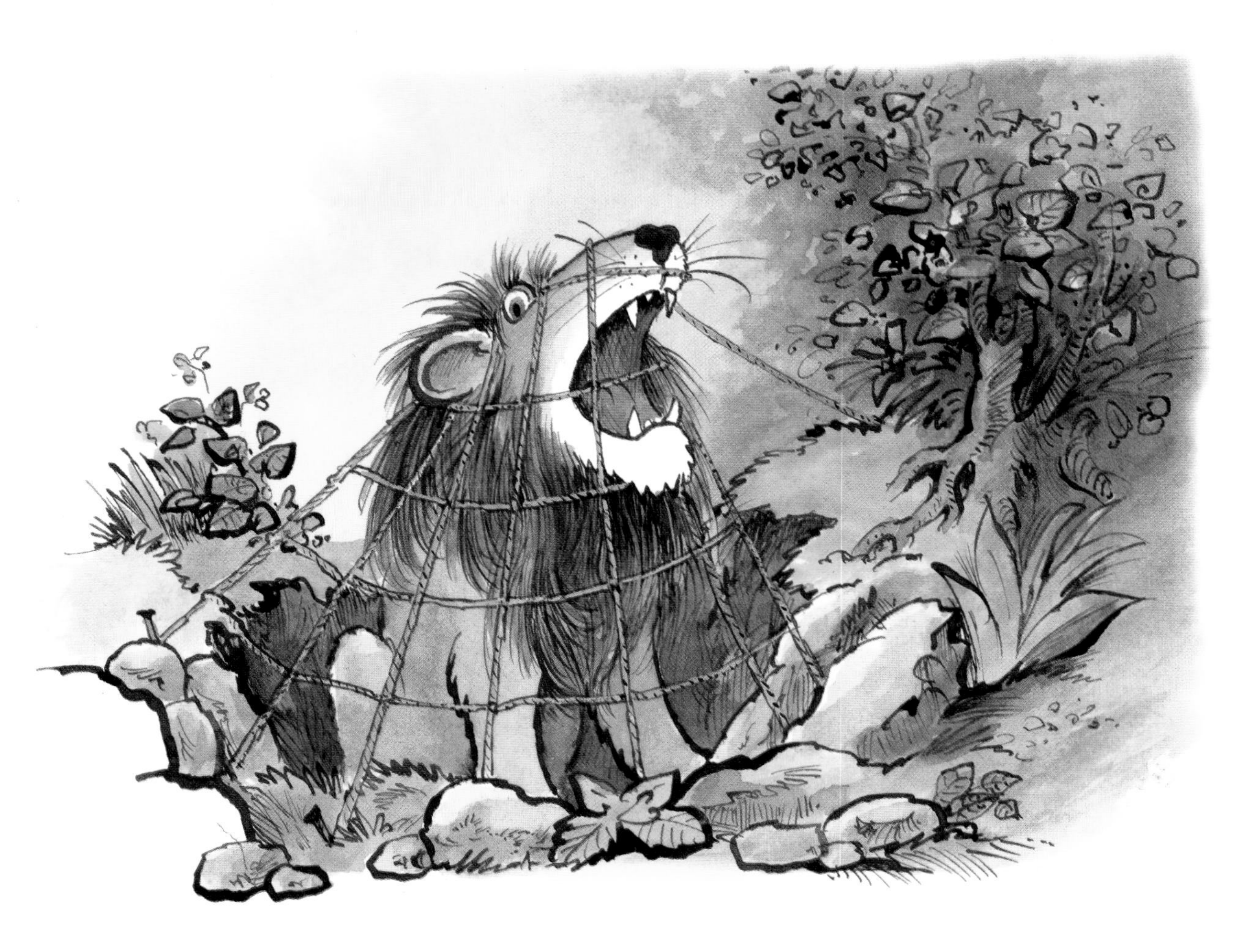

Soon after, the lion was caught in a net. He had been hunting in the forest because by then he really was hungry. He did not know that some men, hunting, had set a trap for him. He roared with anger. It was a frightening sound. All the animals in the forest ran away from the terrible noise, except one.

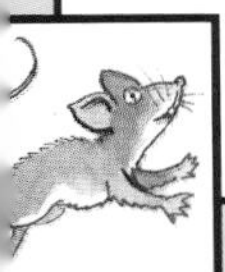
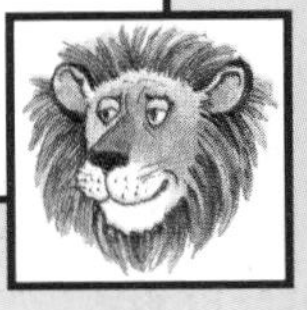

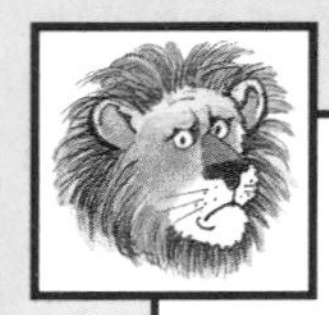

The mouse heard the lion's roar
and ran to help.

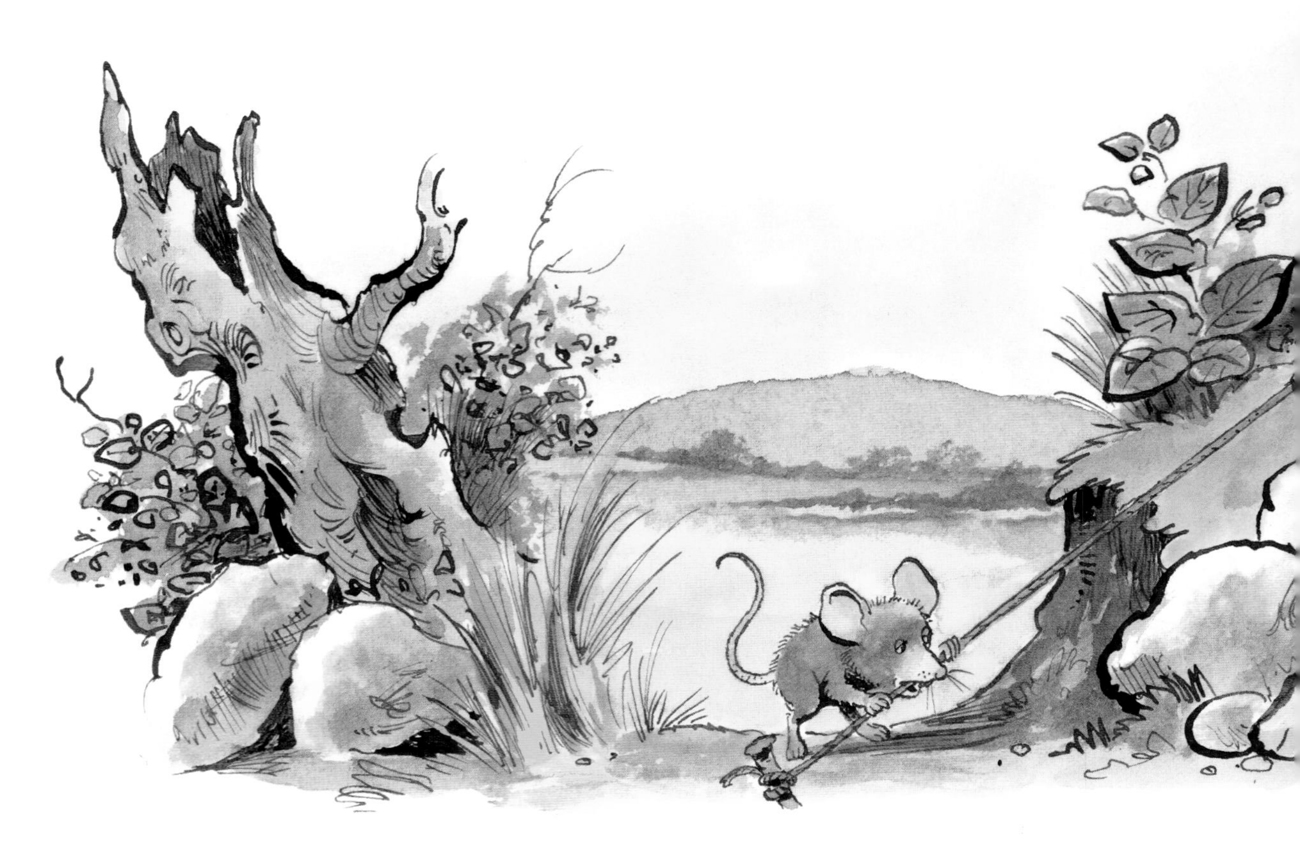

The mouse heard the lion's roar and ran to help.
He knew that the lion was in trouble, and he remembered the promise he had made when the lion had let him go.

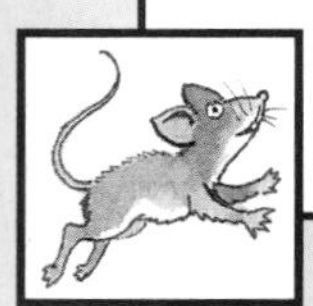

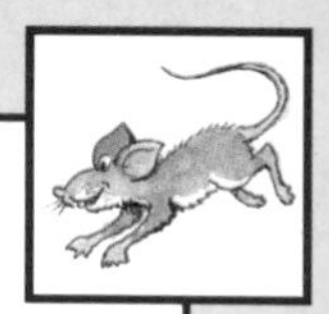

With his sharp little teeth the mouse bit through the net.

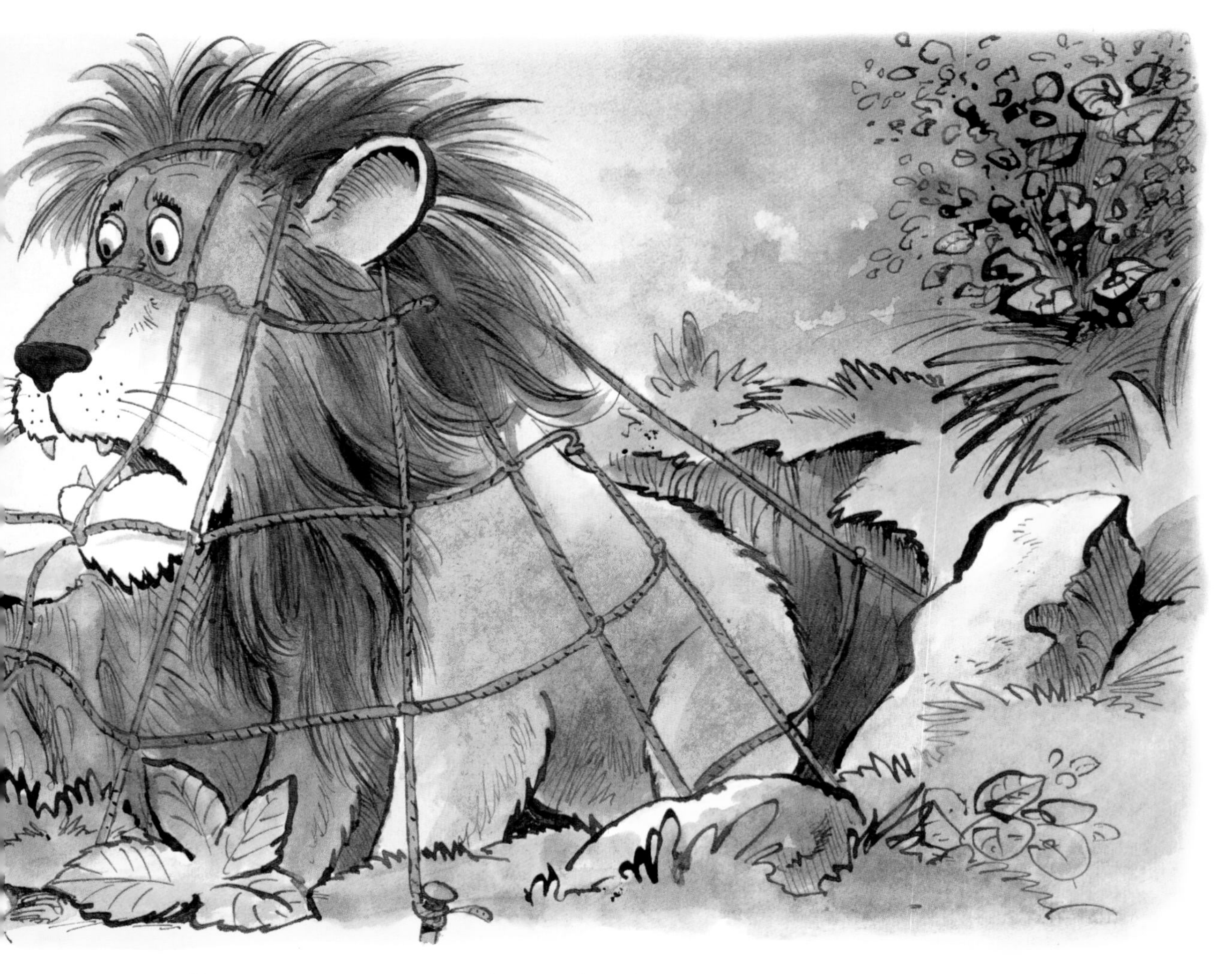

The mouse saw that the lion was caught in a net made of strong ropes. With his sharp little teeth the mouse bit through the net. It was hard work and took a long time but the mouse went on nibbling until at last he made a big hole in the net.

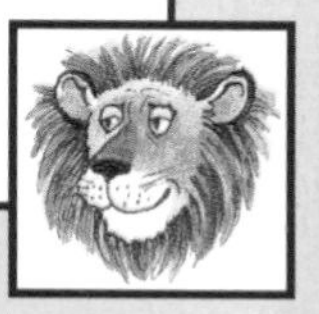

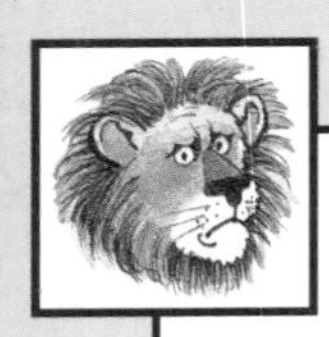
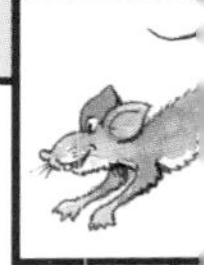

The lion was free!
You see, a mouse *can* help a lion!

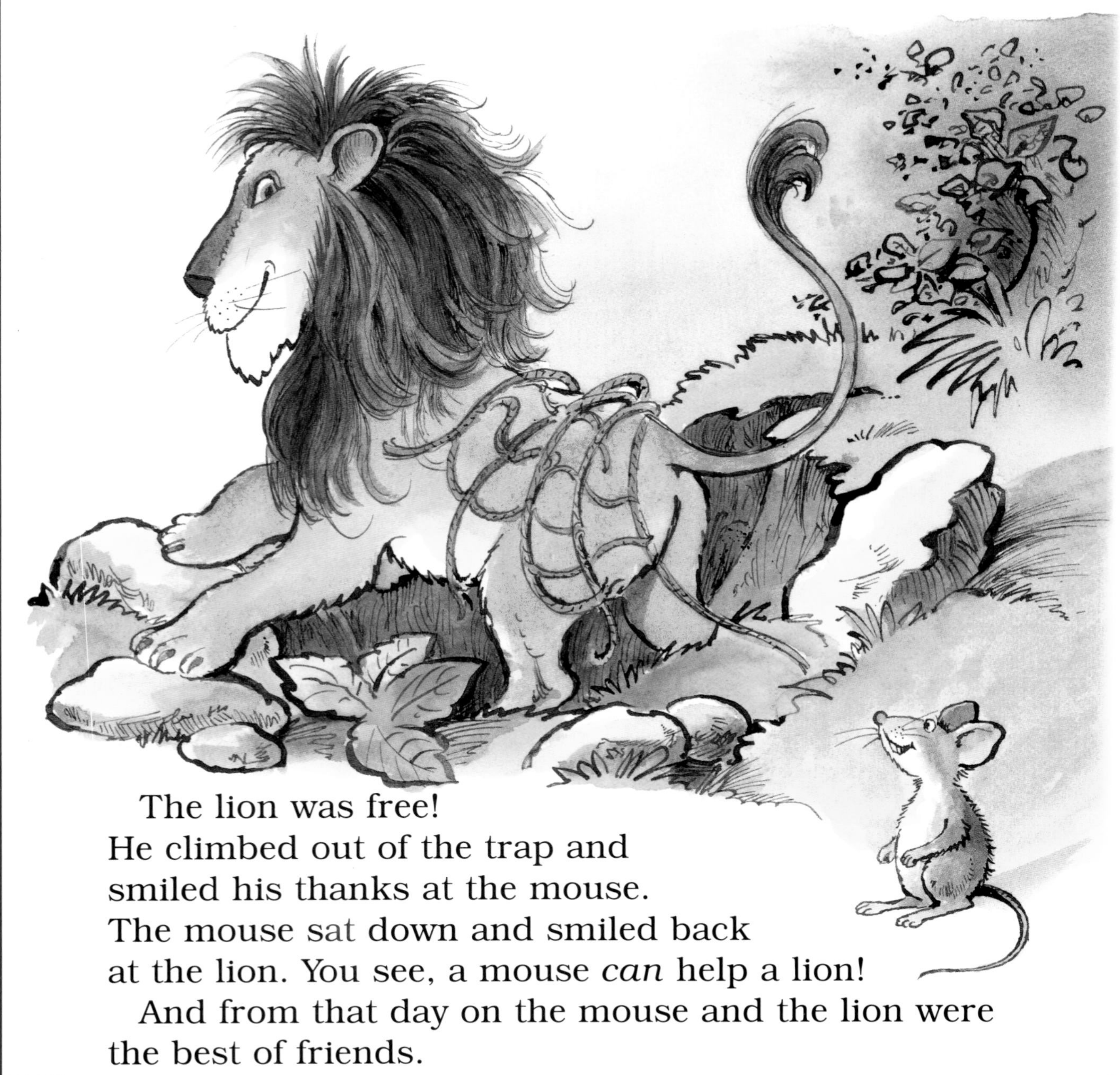

The lion was free!
He climbed out of the trap and
smiled his thanks at the mouse.
The mouse sat down and smiled back
at the lion. You see, a mouse *can* help a lion!

And from that day on the mouse and the lion were
the best of friends.

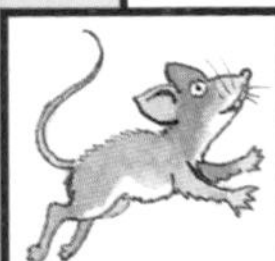
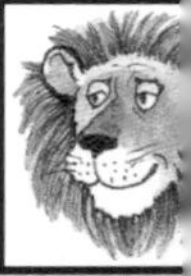